The Sex Toys Guide

A grown up guide for those wanting to know more.

Author: G S Sanders

"The interesting thing is how one guy, through living out his own fantasies, is living out the fantasies of so many other people "

- Hugh Heffner

All Rights Reserved © 2010 G S Sanders

Disclaimer and Terms of Use: No information contained in this book should be considered as health, financial, tax, or legal advice. Your reliance upon information and content obtained by you at or through this publication is solely at your own risk. The author assumes no liability or responsibly for damage or injury to you, other persons, or property arising from any use of any product, information, idea, or instruction contained in the content provided to you through this book.

Table of Contents

	Page
Chapter 1 - Sex Toys Today	1
Chapter 2 - Things to Know About Sex Toys	2 - 3
Chapter 3 – Reasons to Buy a Sex Toy	4 - 7
Chapter 4 - Your First Sex Toy	6 - 10
Chapter 5 - Women's Sex Toy Questions	13 - 14
Chapter 6 - Most Popular Sex Toys	15 - 17
Chapter 7 - Caring for Your Sex Toy	18 - 20
Chapter 8 - Facts About Dildos	21 - 23
Chapter 9 - Facts About Vibrators	24 - 26
Chapter 10 - Facts About Lubricants	27 - 30
Chapter 11 - The Best Materials for Sex Toys	31 - 34
Chapter 12 - Choosing an Anal Sex Toy	35 - 37
Chapter 13 - More on Anal Sex Toys	38 - 40
Chapter 14 – About Cock Rings	41 - 43
Chapter 15 - Cock Ring Tips	44 - 46

Sex Toys Today

Sex toys are now openly discussed. You can buy them in places both on and offline that you'd never have thought possible a few short years ago. Why is this? It can only be that it's now been realised the use of such aids is nothing to be ashamed of.

The liberalisation of the media has had a big role in this. It's quite common to find an actor either referring to a vibrator or even "finding" one for comic effect to the embarrassment of some other character in the show/film or whatever.

You can openly buy them so why not join in with the fun?

This book is intended to provide information on the most popular and commonly available toys.

Have fun!

Three Things You Always Wanted to Know about Sex Toys but Were too Embarrassed to Ask

Am I a pervert if I use sex toys?

No, certainly not. If you could look into the closets and night tables of the nation, you'd be astonished at the high percentage of people who own sex toys. People from all walks of life and all social classes get a kick out of what were once referred to as marital aids. Although individuals with certain religious beliefs may think that sex toys are bad or sinful, many people feel that exploring one's sexuality is a natural and normal part of adult life.

Will sex toys spoil me for "normal" sex?

Absolutely not. If you already have satisfying erotic experiences, including orgasm, then bringing a sex toy into the mix is probably going to enhance your pleasure. Furthermore, if you sometimes have trouble reaching climax, using a toy such as vibrator to heighten arousal may help you to enjoy sexual activity more. And keep in mind, a plastic or rubber device will never take the place of a warm, caring, and sexy partner.

Is everyone going to know I use sex toys?

Not unless you tell them! If you're shy about going into an adult store in your hometown, you can turn to the Internet to find what you need. Look for a store that has been in business for a while and appears to care about customer service. When you shop online, try to buy from a store in your own country. Some erotic supply outlets won't ship across the border because of varying laws and the need to fill out detailed customs forms.

And don't worry what the mail carrier is going to think when he delivers your naughty parcel. Discreet packaging is a hallmark of adult-oriented shops. In fact, sex toys can be obtained in complete privacy. The only tell-tale sign might be the wide smile on your face.

Three Reasons to Buy a Sex Toy (and One Reason Not To)

Sexuality is a natural part of life and so it is not surprising that many of us have a great interest in the subject. Specialty stores carrying an impressive range of sexual aids and accessories are popping up in just about every city and town, not to mention on the internet. Sex toys are popular and gaining mainstream acceptance because they serve many purposes. Here are three good reasons for buying a sex toy and one reason to think twice before you spend the money.

1) Your sex life is getting boring

After you've been with someone for a while, it's easy to slip into a sexual routine where you do the same things every time. You have sex more out of habit than desire. And sometimes you'd rather watch the latest episode of CSI than engage in intimate relations. What you need, whether you realize it or not, is something to jumpstart your stalled love life. Sex toys are an easy and fun way to bring novelty and surprise to the bedroom. They will help you and your partner to experience new sensations and explore your erotic fantasies together.

2) You or your partner has difficulty reaching orgasm

If your partner says it doesn't matter whether she (or he) comes, don't believe it. It does matter. We are all entitled to enjoy sex as much as we can. But many women and a significant number of men sometimes have problems reaching climax. In that case, sex toys are a great tool for increasing arousal and helping things along because they provide an intense or unusual type of stimulation. A mutually satisfying sex life is a significant factor in the long-term success of your relationship. Don't underestimate its importance.

3) You want to enjoy sex without a partner

Most of us have the need and desire to express our erotic nature. Typically we seek out a partner for physical intimacy. But there are times in just about everyone's life when they are alone. You may be single, widowed, divorced, or too busy to pursue a relationship. Fortunately, many toys are great for solitary play.

Of course, a toy isn't exactly a substitute for a warm body, but it's far better than some other options. You don't have to hook up with a stranger just to get a little satisfaction. You don't have to go into unsafe situations or spend too much money hoping for an invitation back to your date's apartment. And believe it or not, even a person in a relationship may enjoy solo play and the freedom to explore his or her own body at leisure.

However, there are times when a sex toy really isn't the solution. For example, don't buy a sex toy to replace your significant other. If you are rejecting the sexual aspect of your relationship and choosing instead to spend time alone with your toy, that's a bad sign. You really need to deal with whatever issues you may be having instead of distancing yourself from your partner.

Sex toys are simply a means to let you express your erotic side in a new way. They are not a magic remedy for all your problems. They can, however, make a dull evening more interesting or promote greater intimacy in a relationship. If you have realistic expectations about what a sex toy can do for you, you'll probably find that the money you spend on toys is some of the best you've ever spent.

Three Tips for Buying Your First Sex Toy

With such a wide array of sex toys and erotic accessories available these days, it can be confusing to sort through all the choices and find the toy that's right for you. There are several important things to consider before you make your purchase, from communicating with your partner to paying attention to quality. Here are three tips to make buying a sex toy a little easier.

1) Involve your partner

If you're in a relationship, you probably intend to use the toy with your significant other. Rather than spring it on an unsuspecting partner – honey, look what I bought! – discuss the purchase beforehand and get your guy's or gal's opinion about what they might like. Do your best to please them and cater to their fantasies. In fact, why not do some browsing in the local adult boutique together? Don't worry; it's okay to giggle when you're checking out some of the astonishing toys you're going to encounter.

2) Try before you buy

If you're completely unfamiliar with the attributes of sex toys, then you might want some hands-on experience before you whip out your credit card. It's hard to get a sense of how the toy works from just a picture. Good adult toy shops will have products out of the package for demonstration purposes, and you're free to look without buying.

Think about the size and shape of the toy in relation to your body or your partner's body and consider the way you intend to use the toy. Turn on powered toys and feel the intensity of the sensation. Pay attention to the sound factor as well. Some toys are very noisy, which might be a problem if the walls in your home are thin. Even if you prefer to buy online, seeing the product up close will help you make a great choice. Whether you buy online or offline, returns of sex toys are usually limited to defective merchandise.

3) You get what you pay for

This is true for almost everything in life and is especially true when it comes to sex toys. Sure, you can readily find cheap toys but they are likely to break quickly or fail to perform as advertised. A shoddy plastic vibrator might be good for a laugh, but it's probably not going to last long or produce the kind of sensations you're looking for.

Sex toys range in price from relatively inexpensive to mind-bogglingly pricey. If you're new to sex toys, look for a product somewhere in the middle price range. Spend enough to get decent quality or you'll be disappointed, but don't invest a lot of money in a toy that you're not positive you will love.

Buying your first sex toy shouldn't be intimidating. This is all about fun, remember. Discuss the subject with your partner and get his or her support. Anticipate how exciting it's going to be when you bring your lovely erotic plaything home. Make a point to look for quality products and use some smart judgment to get the best "bang" for your buck.

Three Questions Women Have About Sex Toys

Your best friend has been bragging non-stop about the fabulous new vibrator she just bought online. It sounds like so much fun that you wonder if you're missing out on something. Women today have an amazing selection of adult toys to choose from, all designed to make sex more creative, exciting, and satisfying. Still, before you go shopping, you want to be sure you're doing the right thing. Here are answers to three questions women frequently have about sex toys.

Will using a sex toy ruin me for regular sex?

You may be concerned that using a vibrator or another sex toy will change you in some way. For example, will you be less interested in sex with your partner? Will using a toy decrease your sensitivity or your ability to achieve orgasm without toys? Fortunately, these are needless worries. Most women say that sex toys only enhance their love life.

An inanimate sex toy can never take the place of a loving and affectionate human partner. In fact, you may discover a new interest in sexual relations because you are getting more enjoyment out of the experience. Furthermore, if you were able to have orgasms before, you will still be able to climax in the same way. What you'll probably find is that sex toys offer new sensations and more prolonged or intense pleasure.

How do men feel about sex toys?

A few men might feel a little insecure about your desire to get a sex toy. It's important to reassure your partner that you are not trying to replace him in any way. After all, buying a toy is a sign that you are thinking about sex and wanting more of it, right? That can only be a good thing from your partner's perspective.

It won't take long for your guy to realize the benefits of sex toys in the bedroom. Women generally need more foreplay than men to get to the same level of arousal. A toy can help turn up the heat very quickly and make his job of pleasing you a bit easier. Men are also very visually oriented and will enjoy the erotic picture of their partner using a toy.

What are the most popular sex toys for women?

Vibrators and dildos are the favorite toys for women. The vibrator's main function is to vibrate and stimulate the clitoris and other erogenous zones. The dildo, on the other hand, is meant for insertion into the vagina to produce a feeling of fullness. Some dildos also stimulate the clitoris and G spot from the inside. Many toys are both vibrator and dildo in one.

It's not a bad idea to start with a simple toy and find out what you like or don't like before you spend a lot of money on a complicated and costly toy. You can find product reviews online that should give you an idea what to expect from a product. Be sure to get a bottle of water-based lubricant when you buy your toy if you don't already have some at home (or make a quick stop at the drugstore). A dollop of lube is recommended for most vibrator use and is practically a necessity when using insertable toys. And don't forget the batteries!

Not too long ago, adult toy stores catered to men and were seen as a bit sleazy. But now that women are enthusiastic buyers of sexual accessories, it's easy to find shops that are bright, pleasant, and staffed with knowledgeable people who are happy to explain how any device works. If you're ready to maximize your sensual pleasure, there is nothing to be afraid of. Haven't you waited long enough to explore the wonderful world of sex toys?

What Are the Most Popular Sex Toys?

Do you find yourself wishing that your love life was a little more interesting? Of course, your partner is a wonderful person, but maybe your intimate moments are getting a little predictable. Just as good food becomes great food with the addition of spices and seasonings, good sex can become even better when you spice it up with a little variety. One of the best ways to get excitement into your sex life is with adult toys. This article will tell you about some popular types of sex toys that can add fun to your lovemaking.

One widely used sex toy is the vibrator. As the name suggests, its purpose is to vibrate or move in a way that stimulates whatever part of the body it comes into contact with. This toy is equally suitable for single people or couples. Not too long ago, most vibrators were long, missile-shaped objects, but these days they come in any shape that fits the contours of the body.

The vibrator is especially popular with women, because it can provide consistent and strong stimulation to the clitoris and surrounding area. For many women, using this toy leads to better and more frequent orgasms than intercourse alone. But vibrators aren't only for female pleasure. Some men also like the pulsing vibration of this device when it is used around their genitals. A vibrator may be enjoyed by itself or in conjunction with other activities.

Another popular sex toy is the dildo. Like the vibrator, a dildo can be used on or by both women and men. Dildos are designed for insertion and thrusting into the vagina or anus and are shaped accordingly. They come in a wide range of sizes and materials. You can find very realistic-looking dildos that strongly resemble a penis, complete with veins and textured skin. Other dildos are more abstract shapes, with gentle curves that may resemble a swimming dolphin or a stylized "S" form. Many dildos are designed to make contact with the female G spot or the male prostate.

One variation on the dildo is the butt plug. A butt plug is not intended for thrusting back and forth. It is held in place by the sphincter and provides erotic stimulation to the prostate and perineum area. Butt plugs are generally shorter than dildos and have a wide base to prevent the toy from getting pushed up too far and becoming unreachable.

Then there are the hybrid toys that are both

vibrator and dildo in one. One such combination toy is known as the rabbit. It got its name from the two little prongs above the main dildo stem (vaguely resembling the ears of a rabbit). The dildo part can be inserted into the vagina while the prongs remain outside in position to vibrate and stimulate the clitoris.

This is just a quick sampling of the many sensual toys on the market. As you can see, there's a whole world of fun and exciting devices available to jazz up sexual activity. Many people like to own several different accessories so they can play according to their mood. Do a little product research and you'll soon be eager to expand your horizons with the perfect sex toy.

Advice on Caring for Your Sex Toy

Now that you've invested some of your hard-earned money in a sex toy, you want to make sure that your new possession lasts and gives you your money's worth. To keep it in good working shape and to protect yourself from health hazards, you must take proper care of your toy. Here are some tips about using, cleaning, and storing sex toys correctly.

Put a condom on toys used for penetration. This often overlooked tip lowers the risk of passing along sexually transmitted infections and reduces clean up effort later. If you share the toy with another person during a lovemaking session, put on a fresh condom first. Always use a condom for toys that are used for both anal play and vaginal play.

Use lubrication. Lube and sex toys go together like peanut butter and jelly. Generous use of a lubricant on dildos and butt plugs makes entry slippery and pleasant and also reduces the chance of irritating delicate membranes.

KY Jelly is perhaps the most widely known lubricant, but there are many others to choose from, depending on your requirements. You can find lube wherever you buy sex toys or pick it up near the condom section in the drugstore. Never use petroleum jelly, cooking oil, shortening, or other food substances for lube as they can cause infections or other problems.

After playing with your toys, take time to clean them up. You certainly don't have to leap out of bed to perform this task; just make sure you wash toys before putting them away. Be sure to read the directions on the package for any special cleaning instructions.

In general, you can clean toys with anti-bacterial soap and warm water, making sure to rinse well. Avoid soaking toys in water for any length of time, and don't immerse battery-operated toys in water or get water in the battery compartment. Dry your toys with a soft towel before storing.

Leather and rubber accessories such as harnesses and masks may be cleaned with soap or leather cleaner on a damp cloth. Follow with a leather conditioner to prevent drying and cracking. If a toy can't be cleaned thoroughly, don't share it with others.

Treat toys with care, especially battery-operated or electric devices, and try not to drop or throw them on the floor or a hard surface.

Store your toy in the original box or in a clean cloth bag, away from light and heat sources. Remove the batteries before putting it away. Keep your plaything (and fresh batteries) in a discreet but handy place so you don't have to go searching for it when you're ready for some fun!

Sex toys can bring a lot of pleasure and excitement to your erotic experiences, so they are worth caring for properly. A little attention to hygiene will protect your health and ensure a long and happy partnership with your favorite toy.

What You Need to Know About Dildos

Mention adult toys and one of the first things to come to mind is probably the ever reliable dildo. Anyone with a genuine interest in sex toys probably has one or more of these tucked away. Some enthusiasts own an impressive collection of sizes, shapes, and colors to match every mood and desire. Let's take a closer look at this popular sex toy and see what makes it such a favorite.

Dildos are objects intended for insertion into the vagina or rectum. They work equally well for solitary play or couples play. Although you may think this toy is specifically for women, that's not really true. Both men and women may enjoy using a dildo for anal penetration. Some couples like to reverse roles with the woman using a dildo on her male partner.

Dildos are often, but not necessarily, shaped like a penis. Some individual appreciate a highly realistic toy. For them, an ultra-detailed silicone model complete with veins and accurately shaped penis head might be just perfect. Other people prefer a dildo that is more abstract in shape and color, and there are plenty of these on the market as well.

Many dildos are curved to reach and stimulate the G spot, which is a sensitive gland located behind the pubic bone in women. Another variation is the double-penetration dildo. This type has a long thick part for vaginal penetration and a shorter, thinner part for anal penetration. Some dildos even contain a vibrating component to provide additional erotic sensations.

The highest quality and most durable dildos are made from silicone rubber. They are also the most costly. If you're not sure what size and shape of toy you prefer, you may want to start off with a less expensive dildo made from jelly rubber or latex rubber. A dildo is generally stiffer and less flexible than a penis, so choose something a little smaller in width than you might think you can handle.

Using lubricant with your dildo will make both vaginal and anal play much more enjoyable. You'll want to pick up a bottle of water-based lube when you buy your toy so you will always have some handy. Don't use silicone-based lube with silicone dildos or you will ruin your toy.

Cleanliness is important for all sex toys, but

especially so for dildos. Be sure to clean your dildo with soap and warm water or toy cleaner when you've finished with it. Materials such as jelly rubber can retain bacteria and be hard to clean thoroughly. It's not a bad idea to put a condom over the dildo before engaging in play.

Experimenting with a new sex toy may be just what you need to perk up your love life. The fun you can have with a dildo is really limited only by your imagination. Pay a visit to your local adult toy store or do a little online shopping. There are so many varieties available that you're bound to find a dildo that tempts you to indulge in a little sensual diversity.

What You Need to Know about Vibrators

As a sex toy, the vibrator is second to none. It's a favorite of many women and is quite possibly the most popular adult toy on the market. The vibrator serves a unique function and there are times when nothing else will do. However, it's also one of those sex toys that can be a thrill or a disappointment. There are so many variations on the basic concept that it can be a real challenge to figure out which one is right for you. Here are some things you should know about vibrators.

A vibrator is used primarily by women for clitoral stimulation. The toy's biggest selling point is that it offers a fairly reliable way for women to achieve orgasm. A vibrator can provide more intense and sustained stimulation than fingers or tongue. Even for women who can easily reach climax in other ways, a vibrator can boost sensation and arousal very quickly. A vibrator can also be used to great effect on the male body. Many toys intended for men now include a vibrating mechanism.

The classic vibrator that most people are familiar with is phallus-shaped, 4 to 6 inches long, and made of plastic or rubber. A popular variation is the clitoral vibrator, which tends to be smaller than the phallus-shaped version and can be egg or bullet-shaped. These also come in animal shapes such as rabbits, bears, cats, or dolphins. The selling points of this type of vibrator are focused, intense stimulation and more precise control of speed and intensity. Then there is the G spot vibrator, which is long and curved to stimulate the G spot from inside the vagina.

Some of the newer vibrators are multi-functional, combining internal G spot stimulation and clitoral stimulation. They may have moving and rotating parts as well as a vibrating component. If you want to go really high-tech, check out the latest vibrator models that contain a micro-processor with programmable vibration patterns.

When it comes to selecting a vibrator, the intensity of the vibration is one of the most important criteria. Electric models are generally more powerful than battery-operated ones. On the down side, they are also more expensive and the cord can be restrictive when you're using the toy. Battery vibrators are more portable and are available in more sizes and styles. You'll find that toys that use C batteries are more powerful than those that run on AA or A batteries. Vibrators can be noisy so if sound level is a concern for you, try out the toy before buying. Hard plastic makes more noise than softer rubber.

How much power you want from your vibrator is a matter of personal preference, but be careful not to buy a toy that is too weak. You can always tone down a vibrator that is too strong by putting a towel or cloth between you and the toy. But a feeble vibrator is just going to be annoying. Online adult toy stores often have customer reviews of their products. These can be a good source of unbiased information and guidance when you are comparing vibrator models.

Fans of adult toys would say that no personal toy collection is complete without a vibrator. This is one sex toy that you may want to spend a little more money on right from the start. The very cheap plastic ones are flimsy and barely worth the effort. Make sure the vibrator you choose has the qualities that are important to you so that you can look forward to many enjoyable hours with your toy.

What You Need to Know about Sex Toys and Lube

When you shop in an adult novelty store, you'll normally see a selection of lubricant lotions prominently displayed alongside the vibrators, dildos, and other goodies. Sex toys are simply more fun when used with lubricant (often referred to as lube). And for some types of play, lube is an absolute must. Let's take a look at why you need to use lube and what type is best for your situation.

A lubricant is basically a liquid or jelly that reduces friction between objects. Of course, products such as KY Jelly are best known as a means to replace or supplement vaginal lubrication during intercourse. But lube is useful for other types of sexual activity, too.

For example, lubricant is used to make inserting a sex toy into any orifice easier and more pleasant. The generous application of lube reduces the risk of damage to delicate tissues in the vagina or rectum. Lube is highly recommended when using a vaginal dildo because the natural lubrication tends to dry out faster than it does during regular intercourse. Furthermore, lube is essential for anal play. Lubricant use doesn't have to be limited to insertable toys, either. Many types of vibrators or masturbation devices feel much nicer when you add a bit of lube.

Don't be stingy with the stuff. Use as much lubricant as you need to make everything slip and slide the way you want it to. Warm the lube in your hand before applying it to body parts. And have a small towel or tissues near by in case things get too messy.

It's important to choose the right type of lube for the activity. The ingredients in some lubes are not compatible with certain toy materials, so make sure you know what is in the bottle. The three main types of lube are water-based, silicone-based, and oil-based.

Water-based lubes have the thinnest consistency and are suitable for most types of sex play. Any toy that can be used with lube can handle a water-based formulation. These lubes are the easiest to clean up and can be quickly washed away with water and maybe a little soap. When you're not sure what product to buy, pick up a bottle of water-based lube.

Silicone-based lubes have an oilier feel than water-based lubes. They have the advantage of being waterproof and can be used in the bath. Some people prefer this type of lube because it lasts longer than water-based lube during play, and it can be revived with a little water if it dries out. Silicone-based lubes are compatible with latex toys or condoms. But they will damage silicone or Cyberskin toys. You can generally keep these toys safe by completely covering the toy with a condom. Clean-up of silicone-based lube requires soap and water.

Finally, there are oil-based lubes, which have the thickest consistency and are perfect for anal play. On the other hand, this type of lube is not recommended for vaginal use because it can cause infections. Oil-based lubes are not compatible with toys or condoms made of latex, so be aware. Wash up thoroughly with soap and water when you're finished.

For health reasons, only lubes made specifically for sexual activity should be used for that purpose. Please don't go scrounging through the kitchen or garage for something slick. You can find safe, quality lubricants at the drugstore or wherever you buy adult toys.

    If you're interested in sex toys, you will definitely have to make friends with lubricant. Remember to pick up a good-sized bottle of your preferred brand when you bring your new toy home. That way you'll be ready for fun whenever the mood strikes you.

Best Materials for Sex Toys

When you go shopping for sex toys, you must realize that most of the time you get what you pay for. Toys vary in quality and workmanship, and some toy materials are more desirable for certain purposes. You probably want to get the best value for what you spend, so you need to understand why some materials are better than others. Here is a guide to the most common materials for sex toys to help you make the best buying decisions.

Most knowledgeable people will tell you that silicone toys are the top of the line. Silicone is highly suitable for sex toys because it is non-porous, hypo-allergenic, and durable. The material is extremely versatile and can be molded into realistic shapes or abstract forms. Toys also come in a rainbow of colors to complement your aura or match your home decor. Silicone is easy to clean, an important selling point for many people. It conducts vibration well and also absorbs and retains body heat. The main drawback may be price - silicone toys are usually more expensive than other toys. But if quality and durability are priorities, you can't go wrong with silicone.

Another widely used material for sex toys is jelly rubber. This substance is flexible but not as smooth or realistic-looking as silicone. Jelly rubber has the primary advantage of being cheap. It does have its drawbacks, though. Jelly toys don't really stand up to long use. The material is semi-porous and can be hard to keep adequately clean. In addition, jelly rubber contains phthalates, which are known to be carcinogenic. Phthalates can also cause an allergic reaction in some individuals. For all these reasons, it's recommended to use a condom over jelly rubber toys.

Latex rubber is the most common material for sex toys. It is widely used because it is cheap and easy to work with, but some people object to the smell of latex rubber and quite a few are allergic to latex. As a result, it is gradually being replaced in the market by newer and less offensive materials. Toys made from latex rubber are not very durable and won't last through years of use. But because such toys are relatively inexpensive, you can experiment with several different styles or sizes of latex toys without emptying your bank account. As a material, latex is porous and not as easy to clean as silicone. Like jelly rubber toys, latex toys are best covered with a condom before use.

Plastic is another widely used and inexpensive material. Plastic is particularly suitable for vibrators because it's durable and conducts vibration well. It's also hard, smooth, and easy to keep clean. However, plastic toys can break if dropped or banged against a hard surface.

Glass and acrylic toys are specialty items that are often valued for their visual appeal as much as their utility. Such toys are designed to be beautiful as well as functional, and they are usually quite expensive. Glass (actually medical-grade Pyrex) and acrylic toys are very hard, very durable, and easy to clean. Metal is another uncommon sex toy material and its use is mostly limited to cock rings, balls, and BDSM accessories.

One of the recent advances in sex toy construction is the invention of material that mimics the feel of human skin and flesh. Toys with this as a component are sold under various tradenames such as Cyberskin, Softskin, or Ultraskin. The material is very soft, elastic, and porous, but because it is so delicate it is rather easy to tear or damage. It's also difficult to clean, requiring a special toy cleaner for the job. Condom use is recommended with these toys to keep them cleaner and help them last longer.

Depending on your needs, you may be just as happy with a cheaper toy as with a high-end version. Just make sure you know what you're getting when it comes to materials and workmanship. That way you will have realistic expectations about how long your toy will last and how easy it will be to keep clean.

What Type of Anal Sex Toy is Right for You?

In the realm of sex toys, anal toys hold a special mystique. Anyone wanting to add a little something extra to their sexual repertoire would do well to consider buying one of these toys. Both men and women interested in trying anal sex play have many options to choose from. To help you decide which anal sex toy is right for you, here is a quick overview of the three main types.

Butt plugs are designed to be inserted into the rectum and remain there during other sexual activity. They produce a feeling of fullness as well as stimulate the sensitive muscles in the anus. Some will also stimulate the male prostate gland. Butt plugs come in a wide variety of shapes and sizes. The dimensions range from "pinky finger" tiny to "you've got to be kidding me" monstrosity. However, when buying your first butt plug, think small. You can always graduate to a larger plug after you've gained some toy experience.

The shape of the plug is probably less important than size but it's still worth considering.

Many toys have a narrow tip, wider middle, and then narrow neck with a wide flared base. Longer models tend stay in better. If the toy is to be used by a man, he may prefer a curved design that stimulates the prostate gland.

Anal dildos are intended for anal penetration and movement. Not all dildos are suitable for anal use. Anal dildos are usually smaller than vaginal dildos. Like butt plugs, they should have a wide base that prevents the toy from going completely inside the rectum. It's best to start with something narrow. Don't get too ambitious right away. There's nothing to prove here. You can have fun with a dildo that's a little smaller than you can easily handle. But a dildo that is too large will just be a waste of money because you won't want to use it. When it comes to size, length is not as significant as width. However, if the dildo will be used with a harness, look for something a bit longer to account for the length lost in the harness.

Anal dildos come in a variety of shapes. Many people prefer toys with a bit of a curve that fits the contour of the rectum. Silicone dildos offer the best quality and widest selection. They are also easy to clean, can be boiled, and last for a long time. However, if you want to start with a less expensive toy, a jelly rubber dildo may work just fine for you. Be sure to cover it with a condom because the material is hard to clean properly.

Anal beads offer an entirely different sensation than plugs or dildos. The toy is, as the name implies, simply a string of beads that is inserted into the anus and then pulled out slowly. This action stimulates the two sphincter muscles in a way that some people find pleasurable. The traditional style of anal beads is a row of plastic or rubber beads tied on a cord. Beads like this are hard to keep clean and really not recommended. Instead, look for a toy that is one molded piece of rubber or silicone shaped like beads on a string. As with most sex toys, silicone is the preferred material because of its durability and ease of cleaning. But for the novice, rubber beads are less expensive and probably a better choice until you are sure you like this type of toy.

Don't be afraid to explore all the erogenous zones of the body. It's easy to keep your sex life exciting and creative as long as you are willing to try something new once in a while. Before you go shopping for toys such as butt plugs, anal dildos, and anal beads, be sure to educate yourself so you bring home the item that is going to provide you with the most rewarding experience.

What You Need to Know about Anal Sex Toys

Anal sex toys inspire a great deal of curiosity and perhaps a little trepidation. Part of their appeal is the sense of venturing into forbidden territory. The anal region of the body is very sensitive, containing a multitude of nerve endings that can give pleasure. Many people are interested in exploring this erogenous zone with adult toys specifically designed for the purpose. Here, for the curious, is an overview of anal sex toys.

By definition, anal sex toys are those made to be inserted into the rectum. This activity produces an erotic sensation that can be very enjoyable, whether the toy is used for solitary play or with a partner. Both women and men of any sexual orientation use these toys. Men have the added bonus of a prostate gland which, when stimulated from inside the rectum by a toy, can greatly enhance the male orgasm.

The basic categories of anal sex toys are butt plugs, anal dildos, and anal beads. Each type is available in almost endless varieties. Butt plugs and anal dildos are similar but have one significant difference. Butt plugs are meant to be inserted and left in place in the rectum for short or long periods of time. Dildos, on the other hand, are intended for movement in and out. Anal beads, as the name suggests, look like a string of beads of the same or graduated size. The beads are inserted and then slowly pulled out when desired.

When it comes to anal toys, safety should be your first consideration. The anus and rectum are composed of delicate tissues that can be damaged if care isn't taken. You should only use toys that are made for anal use. Experimenting with objects you might find lying around the house is definitely not recommended! Toys should be smooth, without sharp edges that can cause harm. They should be made of durable material that is unlikely to break and can be easily cleaned, such as plastic, silicone rubber, or metal. The shape is also important - anal toys should have a wide base that keeps them from slipping all the way inside. You don't want to be forced to make a trip to the emergency room just because you were engaging in a little sex play.

Here are a few more safety tips to keep in mind. The rectum doesn't produce natural lubrication the way the vagina does, so you must always use plenty of lubricant jelly with your toy. Never force anything into the rectum. Slow and gradual opening up of the anus before inserting the toy is essential. If anything hurts, stop what you're doing.

Be sure to keep your toys sparkly clean. Using a condom over a toy can make this job easier. Don't share an anal sex toy with a partner without cleaning it. Don't use the toy in the vagina directly after anal use. Wash it thoroughly first or cover it with a fresh condom to prevent the transfer of bacteria. You get the picture - hygiene is important.

Anal sex toys are widely used by a surprising number of people, and there is really no need to be intimidated by them. In fact, you may find that one of these naughty toys is just what you need to increase your sexual pleasure and add a welcome bit of excitement to your love life.

What You Need to Know About Cock Rings

One of the most widely used sexual accessories is the cock ring. It comes in so many styles that there is something to suit just about every man, no matter what his taste. Some people have the misconception that cock rings are only for men who have trouble getting or keeping an erection. Although it can be useful for that purpose, most guys who wear a cock ring do so because they enjoy the way it feels. If you are not too familiar with this item, here are some things you should know about this popular sex toy.

Not all men like the constrictive sensation of a cock ring. But many do, either as an occasional extra or as a regular part of their sex life. Of course, you're not going to know how you feel until you try it out, so your first ring should be something simple and inexpensive. Don't splurge on the fancy models just yet.

Rubber, metal, and leather are the most common materials for cock rings. You may be better off starting with a simple, flexible rubber ring that is easy to slip over the genitals and also easy to remove quickly. Until you're more experienced with this particular sex toy, avoid the metal rings which are hard or impossible to remove when you have an erection. Leather cock rings look cool but can be a little pricy.

When you are selecting a ring, pay attention to how it is fastened and adjusted. Some rings have snaps or Velcro fasteners. Others have a bead or knot that moves up or down for a tighter or looser fit. Soft rubber rings can be stretched over the penis before or after erection.

The ideal fit for a cock ring is a matter of personal preference. You may prefer a tight cock ring or something with a little give to it. A ring made of soft rubber will feel less constricting than a ring made of rigid rubber, metal, or leather. Regardless of the type, don't wear a cock ring for more than half an hour at a time. If you experience pain or discomfort, remove the ring immediately.

A basic cock ring may be quite enough to keep you happy. If you are feeling adventurous, though, there are many rings that have additional fun features. For example, you may come across complicated-looking objects known as cock and ball rings (or cock and ball splitters). These rings have additional straps attached. The straps go around the balls, separating and pulling on them for a new erotic sensation. Some cock rings are designed to have weights or a leash attached, great for more intense forms of sexual play. And don't overlook the vibrating cock ring, which offers pleasant sensations for both the wearer and his partner during intercourse.

Interestingly, cock rings don't always stay in the bedroom. Sometimes this sex toy is incorporated into offbeat fashion accessories. An observant eye can easily spot rock stars who casually sport this naughty item in public. At first glance, it's just a piece of jewelry or a component on a leather glove. But to those in the know, it's a sly statement about sexuality and individuality.

A cock ring is a powerful symbol of masculinity and potency. Used as a sex toy, it provides a unique type of sensation that can add pleasure and excitement to your sex life. So what are you waiting for? Once you've tried a cock ring, you might wonder how you lived without one.

Tips for Using a Cock Ring

Like many men, you are interested in expanding your erotic pleasure with sex toys. A great choice for just about any guy is the cock ring. In its more basic form, it's simply a ring that fits snugly around the male genitals, enhancing erotic pleasure and performance. The cock ring is the most masculine sexual accessory and it's extremely popular with men of all ages. Here are some tips for getting the most out of a cock ring.

Your choices when it comes to cock rings are many. Styles range from a basic rubber ring to an elaborate design created from leather and metal. A cock ring may come with extra straps to separate and confine the balls. Some varieties have components from which you can hang weights or attach bondage paraphernalia. You can even buy battery-powered rings that vibrate. However, as a first time user, it's best if you choose something simple. As with anything unfamiliar, you may not know whether or not you like the sensation of a cock ring until you try it. Once you've fallen in love with the feeling, you can upgrade to a more deluxe style if you want.

Make sure you know how the ring is supposed to go on. For example, most rings go around both the base of the penis and the scrotum, but some just go around the penis shaft. If you're not sure, ask the store clerk who should be able to explain any intricacies. Don't be embarrassed; she is there to educate customers.

You're probably intending to use the ring with a partner. Even so, it's an excellent idea to get acquainted with your new toy on your own, without the pressure of an audience. You will want to learn how to put the ring on correctly, and even more important, how to remove it quickly. Adjust any snaps or fasteners to get a secure fit. Now, how does it feel? It should be quite comfortable. If the ring pinches or hurts, you're wearing it wrong. Don't assume you need to get used to discomfort - for safety's sake, listen to what your body is telling you.

The next step is to test it in action. Move around with the ring on and see how it changes your stance. Admire yourself in the mirror. It looks pretty cool, doesn't it? Finally, try masturbating to climax. You'll discover that the sensation is quite different when you're wearing a cock ring. Still happy with the way your toy is working out?

Great! Now you're ready to introduce your new toy to your partner.

You might be wondering whether you can wear a condom with a cock ring. If you want to do that, it's best to use the type of ring that fits behind the scrotum. Watch out for any protrusions on the ring that might tear the condom.

By now you should be feeling quite pleased with your new toy. A cock ring is easy to use and feels fantastic if you take the time to do things right. If you haven't bought your ring yet, drop everything and get to the store right now. The only way to really understand the benefits of a cock ring is to try it out for yourself.

Enjoy life! You're only here once!

Made in United States
Orlando, FL
27 August 2024